The Greatest Plant on The Planet

Dexter & Petula Jones

The Greatest Plant on the Planet

Uwriteitpublishing Company
Goldsboro, NC 27534

The Greatest Plant on the Planet by Dexter & Petula Jones
Copyright © 2018 Dexter & Petula Jones

ALL RIGHTS RESERVED

ISBN-13: 978-1725030336
ISBN-10: 1725030330

First Printing—September 2018

This publication is designed to provide information in regard to the subject matter covered. It is published with the understanding that the author is not engaged in rendering legal counsel or other professional services. If legal advice or other professional advice is required, the services of a professional person should be sought.

- These statements have not been evaluated by the Food & Drug Administration. This product information is not intended to diagnose, treat, cure or prevent any diseases.

The Greatest Plant on the Planet

Table of Contents

Acknowledgements

I would like to first off acknowledge the Creator and Maker of all plant life and human life—God Almighty. Whatever mankind thinks he has discovered he has only brought to the surface God's creation and therefore the honor and glory belongs to God Almighty. Moringa Oleifera is God's plant and we're privileged to be able to distribute and sell it to help individuals to meet their health and wellness needs and to get their health back. We acknowledge all our customers that has patronize our business in the past and that will patronize it in the future. God bless you all.

About the Authors

Dexter & Petula Jones is first and foremost Ministers of the gospel of Jesus Christ. Evangelists, that believes in going beyond the church walls to reach the lost with the good news of the gospel. Ministry is their first love because God saved them both out of a world of sin and transformed their lives and made them righteous through Jesus Christ. Now they're going about their Father's business letting the world know that Jesus is the Savior of the world and he came to reconcile man back to God.

Their second love is spreading the good news about God's Superfood Moringa Oleifera. This amazing product has changed their life physically and has enabled them to live a healthy life as well as a life of prevention from sickness and diseases. They know firsthand that the goal is wellness and prevention of disease rather than restoring health to a sick body.

The testimonies that they've seen from

Individuals that have used Moringa Oleifera on a consistent basis are in many instances amazing.

The manner in which God brought his creation into their hands is also amazing. In August of 2016 a friend of Dexter's nephew Jomo Jones whose name is Kelo was in town coming from Charlotte and he brought some Moringa back in town with him. He introduced all of us to the product and made us a bottle of Moringa water. He was very positive about the benefits of the product and what it had done for him and many other individuals whose testimonies he heard. So he gave us a bottle of Moringa water and after drinking it the product gave me instant energy. My response was, **"what is in this stuff?"** Kelo gave us each a sample to take home to continue to try it in order to reap all the benefits of this amazing plant.

As a God gifted researcher I begin to delve into the history of **"Moringa Oliefera"** and the more I researched the more amazed I became. Day by day I was learning new information about a product that I had never heard of before. I became obsessed with learning about this product that had changed the life of so many people. The more I learned the more I wanted to learn because I could not believe that one product could do all this. I have studied many herbs for 30 + years but nothing had even come close to Moringa Oleifera in a single plant.

Other herbs it was necessary in many instances to add many herbs together to get the full effect, Moringa Oliefera however was able to stand alone and yet supply the body with all the essential nutrients. This plant was truly amazing and the more I researched the deeper it got as I learned that over 1300 articles have been written about Moringa Oleifera as well as many books about the veracity of this superfood.

My ultimate conclusion was this is too good to keep to myself. I have to let the world (or at least my world and as my as I could reach) know about this plant that can do so many things but has been hidden for many years. I told my wife that this was more than just a great product that came into our hands, we have to get the word out. So after going through different processes of selling and distributing Moringa Oleifera we decided to make it a real business and formulate all the legalities we needed to establish our own health store called **"Eden Wellness Moringa."** We named it this because we believe that such a tree must have been in the **"Garden of Eden"** when God created his world and placed the man whom he formed. As the scripture states, *"And the LORD God formed man of the dust of the ground, and breathed into his nostrils the breath of life: and man became a living soul. And the LORD God planted a garden eastward in Eden; and there he put the man whom he had formed. And out of the ground made the LORD God to grow every tree (**the Moringa Tree**) that is pleasant to the sight, and good for food; the tree of life also in the midst of the garden, and the tree of the knowledge of good and evil. And a river went out of Eden to water the garden." Genesis 2:7-10a*

This was the beginning of both a

Ministry and Business for us to introduce
Moringa Oleifera to the world.

1

God's Word on Herbs & Dietary

"He causeth the grass to grow for the cattle, and herb for the service of man: that he may bring forth food out of the earth." Psalms 104:14

In the beginning it was the original plan of God for man to have a plant based diet. God's original plan was not for man to be a meat eater but because of the fall of man it was instituted. The scripture states, *"And the LORD God commanded the man, saying, Of every tree of the garden thou mayest freely eat."* Genesis 2:16 Man was supposed to have a consistent diet of plant based eating. Eating plants was designed to give man all the nutrients that he need, plant based eating was man's meat and could provide everything that his body required. It says, *"And God said, Behold, I have given you every herb bearing seed, which is upon the face of all the earth, and every tree, in the* *which is the fruit of a tree yielding seed; to you it shall be for **meat (food).** And God saw everything that he had made, and behold, it was very good. And the evening and the morning was the sixth day."* Genesis 1:29, 31

When Adam and Eve sinned against God by eating of the forbidden tree then they were plunged into dark knowledge and sin entered into the world. Man therefore had to be expelled from the Garden of Eden. *"And the LORD God said, Behold, the man is become as one of us, to know good and evil: and now, lest he put forth his hand, and take also of the tree of life, and eat, and live for ever: Therefore the LORD God sent him forth **from the garden of Eden,** to till the ground from whence he was taken. So he drove out the man; and he placed at the east of the garden of Eden Cherubims, and a flaming sword which turned every way, to keep the way of the tree of life."* Genesis 3:22-24

After the fall man was given permission to eat meat and no longer just a plant based diet. The scripture shows that God gave man permission to eat meat after the flood of Noah's day and man was now able to supplement his plant based diet with meat. It says, *"And God blessed Noah and his sons, and said unto them, Be fruitful, and multiply, and replenish the earth. And the fear of you and the dread of you shall be upon every beast of the earth, and upon every fowl of the air, upon all that moveth upon the earth, and upon all the fishes of the sea; into your hand are they delivered. Every moving thing that liveth shall be meat for you; even as the green herb have I given you all things. But flesh with the life thereof, which is the blood thereof, shall ye not eat." Genesis 9:1-4*

Now that man can eat meat he now eats both meat and plants and is no longer just a plant eater. However, God has told man certain meats to eat that were best for him and meats that were worse off for him. Later in this chapter we will talk about what meats God gave man permission to eat and which to abstain from. At this point man's diet no longer consisted of just a plant based diet. Many times we are encouraged to go strictly vegan or vegetarian or simply plant based eating but is that the healthiest method for mankind. No doubt you can find many books written from the wisdom and knowledge of man that will inform you about eating and living healthy. About all the benefits of plant based eating and the vegan or vegetarian lifestyle. Truly, the majority of what is written is sound and worth taking heed to. The scripture even tells us in Psalms 104:14, *"He causeth the grass to grow for the cattle, and herb for the service (the aid, help, assistance) of man: that he may bring forth food out of the earth."* A plant based diet has so many benefits for the health of man, **however, because of the depletion of the soil today our food does not have all the powerful nutrients that's needed for a healthy body.** Therefore, mankind must use **supplements** to make sure that his body has all the **nutrients essential** for good health and one of the main herbs (plants) or supplements that God has given to mankind today is **Moringa Oleifera,** which we call God's Superfood.

We will delve into why Moringa is the **superfood of all superfoods** and why it's essential to add this plant in your daily life. But to conclude this chapter I want to end it by stating that mankind is limited in his wisdom and knowledge of plant life as well as human lift and because he is not a creator, only a user of the creation, he lacks exact and full knowledge.

When Jesus Christ walked the earth he could have easily told mankind the best plants to eat and what each plant consist of. He could have told us all the nutrients that one would derive from certain plants and the benefits of eating said plants. But if you will notice, even Jesus Christ himself who was God in the flesh was not a vegan and his diet did not consist of just a plant based diet. If a vegetarian or plant based diet was the best method of eating surely God would know and would have instructed Jesus Christ on the healthiest eating method. If the vegetarian plant based diet was the healthiest eating plan then Jesus Christ would have been a vegan, but we know that this was not the case because on many occasions he ate fish. The scripture says, *"And while they yet believed not for joy, and wondered, he said unto them, Have ye here any meat? And they gave him a piece of a broiled fish, and of an honeycomb. And he took it, and did eat before them. Luke 24:41-43* So we know from this scripture that Jesus was neither a vegan nor only consumed a plant based diet.

Not only did Jesus eat fish but he also ate lamb as well. We are also told in the scriptures that during Jesus life on earth he followed the strict laws of Moses which required that the Jews follow a strict dietary observance of only eating **"clean meats"** that God approved, which includes such things as fish, fowl, lamb and bovine just to name a few.

To further show you that Jesus was not a vegan, vegetarian or based his diet on just plant based eating we have the word of God that tells us that Jesus ate the Passover and the Passover consist of eating lamb. The scripture states, *"Speak ye unto all the congregation of Israel, saying, In the tenth day of this month they shall take to them every man a lamb, according to the house of their fathers, a lamb for an house: And if the household be too little for the lamb, let him and his neighbour next unto his house take it according to the number of the souls; every man according to his eating shall make your count for the lamb. And they shall eat the flesh in that night, roast with fire, and unleavened bread; and with bitter herbs they shall eat it." Exodus 12:3-4, 8*

If Jesus was a total vegan or had only a plant based diet and that was the healthiest way to go then why would he feed people fish to eat? This would be hypocrisy to tell someone to do something that you don't do yourself. The scripture says, *"And when it was evening, his disciples came to him, saying, This is a desert place, and the time is now past; send the multitude away, that they may go into the villages, and buy themselves victuals. But Jesus said unto them, They need not depart; give ye them to eat. And they say unto him, We have here but five loaves, and* **two fishes**. *He said, Bring them hither to me. And he commanded the multitude to sit down on the grass, and took the five loaves, and the two fishes, and looking up to heaven, he blessed, and brake, and gave the loaves to his disciples, and the disciples to the multitude.* **And they did all eat**, *and were filled: and they took up of the fragments that remained twelve baskets full.*

We're not saying that you should not be a vegan, a vegetarian nor have a plant based diet, that's entirely up to you but it's not the only healthy way to eat. What we're stating more than anything is that **God is wiser than man** and if he says it's ok to eat **CERTAIN MEATS** then he knows best. Man is the creature and God is the Creator, therefore he knows more about the body of his creation, than Anatomist, Physiologist, Nutritionist, Vegetarianism, Veganism, Philosophers, Scientist, Health Psychologist, Dietitian, Doctors, Etc...

There are certain meats that God stated were ok to eat and certain that he stated to abstain from, I believe that there were two reasons for this. The **first** were religious reasons and the **second** was because of healthy living. God knew that the meat he told the Israelites to abstain from were **unclean and unhealthy**. Here is a brief list of the **clean** and **unclean** animals and we will make the list in accordance with foods most individuals are more familiar with. This list can also be found in Leviticus 11 and Deuteronomy 14.

A LIST OF CLEAN ANIMALS:

The Greatest Plant on the Planet

1. Ox

2. Cattle

3. Buffalo,

4. Sheep,

5. Goat,

6. Deer,

7. Giraffe,

8. Gazelle,

9. Antelope

10. And mountain sheep, just to name a few.

A LIST OF UNCLEAN ANIMALS

1. Pig

2. Camel,

3. Hare,

4. Rock Badger,

5. *Kangaroo,*

6. *Raccoon.*

7. *Camel,*

8. *Bear,*

9. *Elephant,*

10. *Opossum, just to name a few.*

A LIST OF CLEAN BIRDS

1. *Chicken,*

2. *Duck,*

3. *Goose,*

4. *Dove,*

5. *Quail,*

6. *Teal,*

7. *Turkey,*

8. *Pigeon,*

9. *Partridge,*

10. And Pheasant, just to name a few.

A LIST OF UNCLEAN BIRDS

1. Eagle,

2. Ostrich,

3. Penguin,

4. Stork,

5. Vulture,

6. Bat,

7. Hawk,

8. Seagull,

9. Crow,

10. Condor, just to name a few.

A LIST OF CLEAN WATER ANIMALS

1. Bass,

2. Cod,

3. Flounder,

4. Mackerel,

5. Salmon,

6. Sardine,

7. Trout,

8. Tuna,

9. Whitefish,

10. Grouper, just to name a few.

A LIST OF UNCLEAN WATER ANIMALS

1. Catfish,

2. Shark,

3. Squid,

4. Clam,

5. Crab,

6. *Lobster,*

7. *Oyster,*

8. *Scallop,*

9. *Octopus,*

10. *Tilapia,*

11. *Shrimp, just to name a few.*

A LIST OF CLEAN INSECTS

1. *Locust,*

2. *Crickets,*

3. *Grasshoppers, just to name a few.*

A LIST OF UNCLEAN AMPHIBIANS AND REPTILES

1. *Frog,*

2. *Salamander,*

3. *Newt,*

4. *Turtle,*

5. *Alligator,*

6. *Lizard,*

7. *Snake, just to name a few.*

So my conclusion to the whole matter of whether mankind should or should not eat meat is, **God Knows Better Than Man.** Man's wisdom and knowledge is limited, God's wisdom and knowledge is unlimited. Man's wisdom is finite, God's wisdom is infinite. I say once again, man is the creature and God is the Creator, therefore he knows more about the body of his creation, than Anatomist, Physiologist, Nutritionist, Vegetarianism, Veganism, Philosophers, Scientist, Health Psychologist, Dietitian, Doctors, Etc...The scriptures says, *"For as the heavens are higher than the earth, so are my ways higher you're your ways."* Isaiah 55:9

2

The Greatest Plant on the Planet

"And God said, Behold, I have given you every herb bearing seed, which is upon the face of all the earth, and every tree, in the which is the fruit of a tree yielding seed; to you it shall be for meat."

There is a plant or tree called the Morina Oliefera and it's the greatest plant on the planet. You may ask what makes this plant so great. Well, when God created the Moringa Oleifera tree he placed within that tree all the nutrients that our body need in a single plant. There is no other plant on the planet that can assume that right but Moringa Oleifera. It's amazing the nutrients that it contains, Moringa has:

- 3 times the Potassium in bananas.

- 7 times the Vitamin-C as in oranges.

- 25 times the Iron in spinach.

- 4 times the Calcium in milk.

The Greatest Plant on the Planet

- 4 times the Vitamin A in Carrots.

- 46 + Antioxidants

- 36 Anti-Inflammatories

- 90 + Nutrients.

- 18 + Amino Acids

- 8 Essential Amino Acids—the one your body cannot survive without but cannot manufacture on its own.

- 7 times more Vitamin C than Oranges.

- 2 times more Protein than Eggs.

- 10 times more Vitamin E than Nuts.

- **Moringa contains Omega-3, 6, & 9.**

- **Vitamins:** A (Alpha and Beta-Carotene), B, B1, B2, B3, B5, B6, B12, C, D, E, K, Biotin and more.

- **Minerals:** Alanine, Alpha-Carotene, Arginine, Arachidic-Acid, Aspartic-Acid, Behenic-Acid, Beta-Carotene, Beta-Sitosterol, Biotin, Brassicaterol, Caffeoylquinic, Calcium, Campestanol,

Campesterol, Carotenoids, Chlorophyll, Cholesterol, Choline, Chromium, Cobalt, Copper, Cystine, Delta-7 & 14-Stigmastanol, Delta-5- Avenasterol, Delta-7-Avenasterol, EFA Omega 3, EFA Omega 6, EFA Omega 9, Ergostadienol, Fiber, Flavonoids, Fluorine, Folate (Folic Acid), Gadoleic-Acid, Glucosinolates, Glutamine (Glutamic-Acid — Glutathione), Glycine, Histidine, Indole Acetic Acid, Indoleacetonitrile, Iodine, Iron, Isoleucine, Kaernpferal, Leucine, Lignoceric-Acid, Lithium, Lutein, Lysine, Manganese, Magnesium, Molybdenum, Methionine, Myristtc-Acid, Neoxanthin, Niazimicin, Niaziminins A & B, Niazinin A, Niazinin B, Oleic-Acid, Omega 3, Omega 6, Omega 9, Palmitic Acid, Palmitoleic Acid, Phenylalanine, Phosphorus, Potassium, Prolamine, Proline, Protein, Quercetin, Rutin, Sodium, Selenium, Serine, Silicon, Stearic Acid, Stigmasterol, Sulfur, Superoxide Dismutase, Threonine, Tryptophan, Tyrosine, Valine, Vanadium, Violaxanthin, Xanthins, Xanthophylls,

Zeatin, Zeaxathin, Zinc, Ziroconium. All 8 Essential Amino Acids: Isoleucine, Leucine, Lysine, Methionine, Phenylalanine, Threonine, Tryptophan, Valine. 10 Additional Amino Acids: Alanine, Arganine, Aspartic Acid, Cystine, Glutamine, Glycine, Histidine, Proline, Serine, Tyrosine. Other Beneficial Nutrients: Chlorophyll, Carotenoids, Cytokinins, Plant Sterols, Polyphenols, and more. **All in 1 plant.**

There is no other plant on the planet that can give your body all these **nutrients in 1 single plant.** Many times we experience various sickness and diseases because we are deficient in vitamins and minerals. When you're lacking essential nutrients then your body begins to work against you instead of with you. Let's look at some examples of diseases and deficiencies that can add to these diseases.

HIGH BLOOD PRESSURE: Take for example a person that has high blood pressure they're deficient in such nutrients as: **Potassium, Magnesium, Omega 3 fats, Calcium and Coenzyme Q10 that acts as an antioxidant in our cells,** just to name a few. But if you will notice from the list of nutrients contained in Moringa Oleifera it has all these nutrients in this 1 plant.

ARTHRITIS: A person that has arthritis is deficient in such nutrients as: **Vitamin D, Folate, Calcium, and Omega 3 fatty Acids,** just to name a few. Also, if you will notice that Moringa Oleifera has all these essential nutrients in this one plant.

DIABETES: A person that has diabetes is deficient in such nutrients as: **Vitamin B12, Vitamin D, Vitamin E, Magnesium, Zinc, Vitamin B6, Folate, Vitamin C and Antioxidants,** just to name a few. However, if you will notice from the list of nutrients in Moringa Oleifera all these are contained in this 1 plant.

HIGH CHOLESTEROL: A person that has high cholesterol is most of the time deficient in such nutrients as: **Vitamin B12, Iron, Biotin, Inositol, Chromium, Copper, Manganese, Potassium, Vanadium, and Zinc,** just to name a few. However, if you will notice from the list of nutrients in Moringa Oleifera all these are contained in this 1 plant.

DEMENTIA: A person that is dealing with Dementia is deficient in such nutrients as: **Vitamin B1, Vitamin E, Phosphatidylserine (PS) (is a phospholipid-a fat containing phosphorus), Vitamin B12, Folate, Zinc,** just to name a few. But if you will notice from the list of nutrients in Moringa Oleifera all these are contained in this 1 plant.

FATIGUE (Tiredness or lack of Energy): A person that is experiencing fatigue or lack of energy is deficient in such nutrients as: **Vitamin B12, Folate, Vitamin D, Iron, Magnesium, and Potassium,** just to name a few. But if you will notice from the list of nutrients in

Moringa Oleifera all these are contained in this 1 plant.

CARDIOVASCULAR DISEASE: A person that's experiencing cardiovascular disease is deficient in such nutrients as: **Vitamin D, Coenzyme Q10, Iron, Vitamin B1(Thiamine), Amino Acids, Folate, Flavonoids, Vanadium, Vitamin E,** just to name a few. But if you will notice from the list of nutrients in Moringa Oleifera all these are contained in this 1 plant.

DEPRESSION: A person that's experiencing depression is deficient in such nutrients as: **Omega-3 Fatty Acids, Vitamin D, Magnesium, Vitamin B Complex, Folate, Amino Acids, Iron, Zinc, Iodine, Selenium,** just to name a few. But if you will notice from the list of nutrients in Moringa Oleifera all these are contained in this 1 plant.

HEADACHES: A person that's experiencing various kinds of headaches from migraine to regular headaches are deficient in such nutrients as: **Vitamin D, Riboflavin, Coenzyme Q10, Folate, Vitamin B Complex, Vitamin E, Magnesium, Iron,** just to name a few. But if you will notice from the list of nutrients in Moringa Oleifera all these are contained in this 1 plant.

FIBROMYALGIA: A person that's experiencing fibromyalgia is deficient in such nutrients as: **Vitamin D, Magnesium, Iron, Amino Acids, Vitamin B12, and Calcium,** just to name a few. But if you will notice from the list of nutrients in Moringa Oleifera all these are contained in this 1 plant.

HYPOTHYROIDISM: A person that's experiencing hypothyroidism is deficient in such nutrients as: **Iodine, Vitamin B Complex, Selenium, Zinc, Vitamin D, Tyrosine, Vitamin A, Iron,** just to name a few. But if you will notice from the list of nutrients in Moringa Oleifera all these are contained in this 1 plant.

WEIGHT LOSS: When dealing with obesity or overweight you need to make sure that you're getting the essential nutrients for your physical body. Weight loss is more than just losing weight; you want to make sure that you're healthy while losing that weight. Research has proven that individuals that obtain the lowest amount of nutrients are gaining the most weight. Most individuals are deficient in such nutrients as: **Iron, Vitamin D, Vitamin B Complex, Magnesium, Vitamin A, Iodine, Vitamin C, Calcium,** just to name a few. But if you will notice from the list of nutrients in Moringa Oleifera all these are contained in this 1 plant.

CANCER: A person dealing with cancer has a broader spectrum of things going on but making sure that your body has the essential nutrients can play a great part in recovery. Some research has also revealed that certain forms of cancer are more widespread among some regions where there is great nutrient deficiency.

Some of the nutrients you will need to include in your daily diet are: **Vitamin D, Vitamin K, Iodine, Magnesium, Selenium, Vitamin B Complex, Vitamin C, Iron, Folate, Vitamin A, Coenzyme Q10,** just to name a few. But if you will notice from the list of nutrients in Moringa Oleifera all these are contained in this 1 plant.

While your body is supplied with all the nutrients to combat these diseases you're also taking in an awesome supply of such things as:

- **46 + Antioxidants**

- **36 Anti-Inflammatories**

- **Moringa contains Omega 3, 6, & 9.**

- **18 + Amino Acids**

- **8 Essential Amino Acids—the one your body cannot survive without but cannot manufacture on its own.**

- **Moringa contains Silymarin an Antioxidant that's great for liver problems.**

- **Moringa contains ZEATIN, which regulates cell division and growth, plus it has ant-aging properties that delay cell aging. The ZEATIN in Moringa has several thousand times more in it than any other plant on the planet.**

Moringa is the most powerful superfood that God has ever allowed man to discover to date. It is one product that contains no fillers, additives, preservatives, etc.… Therefore, when you have Moringa you have one natural supplement that covers many things your body requires and needs instead of buying several supplements that can be very expensive. There is no other plant on the planet that carries a more compacted profile of nutrients in one product.

Even if you're eating a properly balanced meal your meal is still deficient in vitamins and minerals because our soils today are depleted by the rigorous growth methods that cause our food to lack the essential nutrients needed for our bodies. Yet, Moringa is the only plant that can provide your body with all the nutrients that's needed on a daily basis. Moringa Oleifera is often called "The Miracle Tree" because of the enormous health benefits that one derives from using it. This plant has a long history of success according to India's age old tradition known as Ayurveda for centuries, used Moringa Oleifera as a healing plant.

Our Moringa sold and distributed at "Eden Wellness Moringa" is superior quality, superior grade, organically grown, 100% pure, non-polluted, high potent, USDA Organic, caffeine free, non-gmo, gluten free, all natural, chemical free & pesticide free. We have the finest leaves, flowers, seeds, etc. harvested in the right stage.

So you see why Moringa Oleifera is called the greatest plant on the planet because no other plant can give your body what it needs in 1 plant. **Knowledge is a powerful thing.**

3

Why Moringa Oleifera

"There is no money in treating healthy people from a physician standpoint." D.L.Jones

Moringa is the most powerful superfood ever discovered by mankind. For thousands of years it has been a remedy for mankind as far back as the Ayurvedic medicine one of the world's oldest medical methods that originated in India over 3,000 years ago and still practiced today. Our objective in bringing to the forefront Moringa in our Western society is to inform individuals of the benefits that are derived from the consumption of this amazing plant. It is a plant that supplies our bodies with all the essential nutrients for a healthy body. This eliminates the widespread cost of having to purchase various supplements to provide your body with the necessary nutrients for wholeness and wellness.

One can spend a small fortune trying to purchase various vitamin supplements to make up the whole of what's needed for a daily supplement. However, with Moringa you have it all in 1 plant.

We encourage individuals to take Moringa for 2 reasons:

1. *Prevention of sickness and disease.*

2. *Restoration of your body to meet your health and wellness needs.*

These are the main reasons why one would add Moringa Oleifera to their daily dietary supplement. We will delve into these two reasons and how God's Superfood can aid, help, and assist mankind in keeping his temple (body) in tip top shape or restoring it to a healthy state. There is no reason why you have to live a life of sickness and disease when God's has already supplied mankind with the remedy for good health. Mankind just has to be obedient to learn and apply what God says about Moringa and how he designed this plant to help our bodies rid itself of toxic things that can hurt us. As well as how Moringa can supply our bodies with the essential nutrients to maintain good health and help reverse bad health.

PREVENTION OF SICKNESS
AND DISEASE

Seeing a sick body restored back to health is a wonderful thing. However, what's better than restoration is a body that remains healthy consistently. No one wants to encounter sickness even if good health or healing is right around the corner. The best method is **PREVENTION** at all cost. One of the great things we've found about Moringa is that it has within it what it takes to get and maintain a **HEALTHY BODY**. Moringa is the greatest weapon against prevention of sickness and disease.

Having Moringa in your system is like always having a doctor on hand because once it gets in your system it works around the clock 24/7 and 365 days a year.

With all the nutrients in Moringa it has been discovered that this amazing plant has the highest protein ratio of any plant analyzed so far. With such inherited protein it's an absolute that your body will not only survive but thrive as every cell in your body is impacted with the highest protein available today in plant form. Because our bodies use protein to repair and build tissue Moringa is an important building block of our body functions. With such an infusion of essential proteins your body will take care of itself as Moringa both prevent the occurrence of disease as well as slow down the rate or frequency of disease.

Moringa is a product when used on a consistent basis has the power to intervene and deter any evidence of disease or sickness. It has the ability to eliminate problems at the source, thereby preventing the occurrence on an issue. Moringa's aim is to empower your body to be able to sustain itself and thereby reduce the risk of developing diseases.

A healthy body honors and glorifies God; a sick body deprives you of use and dishonors God. The scripture says, *"What? know ye not that your body is the temple of the Holy Ghost which is in you, which ye have of God, and ye are not your own? For ye are bought with a price: therefore glorify God in your body, and in your spirit, which are God's"* 1 Corinthians 6:19-20

The key to a healthy life is PREVENTION not RESTORATION. The act of restoration only comes because you have failed in prevention. The one way to prevent diseases is by maintaining good health and keeping a proper assessment of what is going on in your body. **Moringa Oleifera does this for you.**

RESTORATION OF THE BODY TO HEALTH AND WELLNESS

In our society we have millions of individuals that are suffering with various diseases and sickness. From high blood pressure, diabetes, cardiovascular disease, obesity, fatigue, etc.… and it's taking its toll on our society. Individuals that are dealing with these diseases have one thing in mind and that is either healing for their body or restoring their body back to health.

Restoration is needed when you have failed at prevention and now you need to get your body back to health. Well, Moringa Oleifera is also an excellent restorer to health by resupplying your body with the essential nutrients that it has been deprived of and thereby sickness has taken the advantage of your deprivation. There is no need to give up all hope and throw in the towel; Moringa is here to rescue you as God's Superfood.

The Greatest Plant on the Planet

Moringa Oleifera can aid and assist you to return your body to a normal or healthy condition as God designed it to do. Moringa gets to the source of the problem and helps your body to heal itself as the missing nutrients helps your body to fight off toxins that make it sick while at the same time strengthening your body functions by giving it new life as you absorb the miracle working power of Moringa.

There are several ways Moringa does this to help restore health and wellness to your body.

1. *It detoxifies your body.*

2. *It removes the parasites out of your body.*

3. *It builds up your immune system.*

4. *It fights off free radicals with its rich amount of antioxidants.*

5. *It reduces inflammation in the body.*

6. *It protects the cardiovascular system.*

7. It helps to support the brain health.

8. It helps to protect the liver.

9. It helps to protect the kidneys.

10. Moringa contains antimicrobial and antibacterial properties.

11. Moringa helps to reduce stress.

12. It helps to support a healthy digestive system.

13. It helps to maintain strong and healthy bones.

14. Moringa helps to balance your hormones.

15. Moringa protects and nourishes the skin.

16. Moringa contains 90+ nutrients to meet your physical needs.

17. Moringa contains 36 anti-inflammatory compounds.

18. Moringa contains 46 antioxidants.

19. *Moringa contains 8 essential amino acids which your body needs but cannot produce.*

20. *Moringa contains phytonutrients like zeatin, quercetin, beta-sistosterol, caffeeoylquinic acid and kaempferol.*

21. *Moringa boosts energy level naturally.*

Moringa is known by over 100 names in various parts of the world and is now becoming very popular in the United States. In 2008, the National Institute of Health called Moringa Oleifera the **"plant of the year."** Also, according to the ORAC, Moringa scored 157,000, topping all the other antioxidants superfoods on the market today. Including such superfoods as Acai berries, Green tea, Blueberries, Dark Chocolate, Garlic, Goji berries, Pomegranates and Red Wine.

There is no better and more qualified plant today for Prevention or Restoring your health back to normal. Prevention is the key and Restoration is both a process and a journey and Moringa Oleifera is God's Superfood that will bring life back into your body.

4

The Vitamin Myth

"Vitamins are not real they're imitations of the real and just perpetrating the real."

Most vitamins are synthetic or chemical based so therefore you're not getting what you need when taking vitamins. Billions of dollars are spent every year on synthetic vitamins with the hope that these supplements will supply the body with what it needs. However, the truth of the matter is that these synthetic and chemical based vitamins that you're purchasing from your local or chain health stores is really a waste of your hard earned money.

Society is been sold a myth in the vitamin world but the truth of the matter is that synthetic vitamins do not actually improve your health. According to studies there is next to no health benefits in taking store bought vitamins. Yet, millions of individuals are taking vitamins in order to build up their health and so that they will not be deficient in nutrients. The big pharmaceuticals companies are mainly the producers of these manufactured chemicals. These synthetic vitamins in the long run do your body more harm than good. They contain various additives, preservatives, fillers which can actually be harmful or toxic for your body.

Some of the harmful things you will find in these synthetic chemical based vitamins are:

1. *Calcium Carbonate*

2. *Polyethylene Glycol*

3. *Hydrogenated Oil*

4. *Cyanocobalamin*

5. *Food Dye Yellow 6*

6. *GMO Corn Starch*

7. *Titanium Dioxide*

8. *Cupric Oxide*

9. *Artificial Sweeteners (Aspartame)*

10. *Zinc Oxide*

11. *Lactose*

12. *Sugar (Sucrose)*

13. *Food Dye Blue 2*

14. *Soy Lecithin*

15. *Vitamin B6 (Pyridoxine) Pyridoxine Hydrochloride*

16. *Magnesium Stearate*

17. *Artificial Colors*

18. *Artificial flavors*

19. *Mono-and Diglycerides*

20. *Maltodextrin and ascorbic acid, just to name a few.*

Don't fall for the LIE of these big pharmaceutical companies that's distributing these vitamins to some of the most popular stores in America. Vitamin companies say that they making you healthy but it's just another marketing tool to get you hooked on synthetic chemical based vitamins. Look on the back of your vitamin bottle and see if any of the items listed are there? Take the initiative to look up some of the ingredients listed on your vitamin bottle and you will be amazed at what you've been putting in your body under the guise of healthy and natural.

Some people take 10, 15 or more vitamins a day in order to supplement their diet and to eradicate nutrition deficiency. Since the foods we eat today do not contain the nutrients that it use to individuals are consumed with taking vitamins even if they have to take 10 or more a day.

The kinds of vitamins you want to take are not synthetic vitamins but plant based whole food vitamins. Sometimes plant based whole food vitamins can be more expensive but they are worth it for your health. Moringa Oleifera is a plant based vitamin that contains what your body needs from a whole food source and the beauty of Moringa is that you don't have to buy several different vitamins to get what your body need. This 1 plant Moringa Oleifera contains it all.

5

A Deficiency of Vitamin and Mineral

"People are not looking for good health; instead they're looking for a Quick Fix."

Are you constantly been plagued with sickness and diseases?

Do you catch a cold a certain time every year?

Does sickness or disease seem to be a constant occurrence with you?

Many of the problems that plague mankind today can be summed up as a result of a deficiency of vitamins and minerals. Vitamins and minerals play the role of essential nutrients in our body and a continual supply is needed on a daily basis. When God created mankind the foods that he was supposed to eat were designed to infuse his body with the essentials needed to sustain them. The scripture says, *"Behold, I have given you every herb bearing seed, which is upon the face of all the earth, and every tree, in the which is the fruit of a tree yielding seed; to you it shall be for meat." Genesis 1:29"* Every tree in the garden Adam and Eve could eat of and these trees were full of life and would continually provide their body with the essential nutrients. There were no death in the plants or trees only life and the vitamins and minerals contained therein were on a different level than vitamins and minerals today.

God designed the trees to be eaten not just to be admired, the scripture says, *"And the Lord God planted a garden eastward in Eden; and there he put the man whom he had formed. And out of the ground made the LORD God to grow every tree that is pleasant to the sight, **and good for food**."* *Genesis 2:8-9* When something is eaten it's to provide our bodies with the power needed to sustain life by supplying it with the essential nutrients vital for substantiation. The trees were for food and food provides the necessary vitamins and minerals for life, health and strength. When Adam and Eve ate of the trees in the garden their bodies were rejuvenated just like our bodies are when we eat food.

The plants and trees had all the essential vitamins and minerals needed to sustain Adam and Eve's body on a daily basis. The vitamin and minerals in the plants and trees were equivalent to the physical body they possess. A body teeming with life and vitamins and minerals engrafted in the plants to meet the need of such an empowered body. They had to eat for their body sake. Their body needed food and the food provided the nutrients.

As long as they did not eat of the tree of *"the knowledge of good and evil"* they could have continued their existence in perfect health. Their spirts would have been sustained by God spiritually and their bodies sustained by the food that provided the essential nutrients that God provided through the plant and trees. Perfect health on a continual basis, they never knew the devastating effects of such diseases on their physical body as:

- **High Blood Pressure**

- **Diabetes**

- **High Cholesterol**

- **Arthritis**

- **Dementia**

- **Fatigue**

- **Cardiovascular Disease**

- **Depression**

- **Headaches**

- **Fibromyalgia**

- **Hypothyroidism**

- **Obesity or Weight Gain**

- **Cancer**

- **Kidney Disease**

- **Liver Disease**

- **Asthma**

- **Constipation**

- **COPD**

- **Erectile Dysfunction**

- **Epilepsy**

- **Ulcerative Colitis**

- **Hormonal Imbalance**

- **Hepatitis C**

- **Sinusitis**

- **Bronchitis**

- **Psoriasis or Eczema**

- **Or Hundreds of Other Diseases...**

These diseases only came when they disobeyed God and ate of the forbidden fruit. Their physical bodies were no longer teeming with life; it was now on the road to death. The plants and trees were cursed and they lost their vitality and now death was all around. The scripture says, *"And unto Adam he said,*

Because thou hast hearkened unto the voice of thy wife, and hast eaten of the tree, of which I commanded thee, saying, Thou shalt not eat of it: **cursed is the ground for thy sake;** *in sorrow shalt thou eat of it all the days of thy life;* **Thorns and thistles shall it bring forth to thee; and thou shalt eat the herb of the field."** Genesis 3:17-18

The Garden of Eden (the place of paradise) plants and trees full of lively nutrients was no longer the home of God's first man. *"So he drove out he man; and he placed at the east of the garden of Eden Cherubims, and a flaming sword which turned every way, to keep the way of the tree of life."* Genesis 3:24

Now man is in a dilemma because the ground is now cursed and thorns and thistles are now growing up representing death and decay. His physical body has taken a turn for the worse but it could still be sustained to a point by the fact that they could *"eat the herb of the field." Genesis 3:18b* Sickness and disease came as a result of man's separation from God, spiritual death was first and physical death followed. The door to sickness and diseases were now opened wide and sin was the cause which brought separation from God. *"Wherefore, as by one man sin entered the world, and death by sin; and so death passed (physical as well as sickness and disease) upon all men, for that all have sinned." Romans 5:12*

The remedy that God provided for sin is Jesus Christ and the remedy that God has provided for man's physical body to work at an optimum is the *"herb of the field." Genesis 3:18b* Why the herb of the field? The herb of the field has been designed to give mankind the essential nutrients for health and wellness.

"He causeth the grass to grow for the cattle, and herb for the service (aid, help, assistance) of man: that he may bring forth food out of the earth." Psalms 104:14

When mankind uses these God given herbs to provide his body the essential nutrients then his body will not be deficient in vitamins and minerals and the result of non-deficiency is health and wellness. You can abstain from sickness. You can get well. If you will just take the initiative to supply your body daily with the essential vitamins and minerals it needs. There is no need for the powerful vitamins and minerals that were in the plants and trees in the Garden of Eden (our sinful bodies couldn't sustain them), but the nutrients today are equivalent for our bodies today.

However, we will not find the equivalent nutrients needed in **synthetic chemical based vitamins** as stated in the former chapter. They must be **plant based whole food supplements.** There are many plants that God has created to assist and aid our bodies, the only drawback is that until the discovery or shall I say appearance of Moringa Oleifera we've had to join many supplements together to get a whole.

The sickness and diseases that you're experiencing is a result of "**A Deficiency of Vitamin and Mineral.**" When your body does not have the nutrients that it needs then it cannot function as it should. Your body becomes deficient in vitamins and minerals when it doesn't obtain or absorb the amount of vitamins and minerals it requires. Your body must have different amount of each vitamin and mineral in order to stay healthy and when the required amount is not there then you've become deficient in those vitamins and minerals.

In chapter 2 we named out a list of diseases and the deficiency of vitamins and minerals that contribute to these diseases. In this chapter we will list more for your edification and understanding. Here is a list of more diseases and the deficiencies that contribute to these diseases:

ASTHMA: A person that has asthma is deficient in such nutrients as: **Vitamin D,**

Vitamin E, Vitamin C, Polyunsaturated fatty acids (Omega 3 & 6), Selenium, Zinc, Magnesium, Manganese, Flavonoids, Vitamin B12, Folate, Vitamin B6, just to name a few. But if you will notice from the list of nutrients contained in Moringa Oleifera it has all these nutrients in this 1 plant.

ERECTILE DYSFUNCTION: A person that is experiencing erectile dysfunction is deficient in such nutrients as: **Vitamin D, Manganese, Magnesium, Vitamin B3, Folate, Vitamin B12, Amino Acids, Zinc,** just to name a few. But if you will notice from the list of nutrients contained in Moringa Oleifera it has all these nutrients in this 1 plant.

KIDNEY DISEASE: A person that's experiencing kidney disease is deficient in such nutrients as: **Vitamin B Complex, Iron, Vitamin D, Vitamin C, and Calcium,** just to name a few. But if you will notice from the list of nutrients contained in Moringa Oleifera it has all these nutrients in this 1 plant.

LIVER DISEASE: A person that's experiencing liver disease is deficient in such nutrients as: **Antioxidants, Zinc, Selenium, Beta-carotene, Vitamin D, Vitamin A, and Magnesium,** just to name a few. But if you will notice from the list of nutrients contained in Moringa Oleifera it has all these nutrients in this 1 plant.

EPILEPSY: A person that's experiencing epilepsy is deficient in such nutrients as: **Vitamin B6, Calcium, Carnitine, Vitamin D, Vitamin E, Folate, Magnesium, Selenium, Vitamin B1, Vitamin B12, Sodium,** just to name a few. But if you will notice from the list of nutrients contained in Moringa Oleifera it has all these nutrients in this 1 plant

ULCERATIVE COLITIS: A person that's experiencing ulcerative colitis is deficient in such nutrients as: **Vitamin B12, Iron, Vitamin D, Vitamin K, Folate, Selenium, Zinc, Vitamin B6 and Vitamin B1,** just to name a few. But if you will notice from the list of nutrients contained in Moringa

Oleifera it has all these nutrients in this 1 plant.

GOUT: A person that's experiencing gout is deficient in such nutrients as: **Calcium, Vitamin D, Potassium, and Magnesium,** just to name a few. But if you will notice from the list of nutrients contained in Moringa Oleifera it has all these nutrients in this 1 plant.

HORMONAL IMBALANCE: A person that is experiencing hormonal imbalance is deficient in such nutrients as: **Vitamin C, Vitamin E, Calcium, Magnesium, Vitamin B Complex,** just to name a few. But if you will notice from the list of nutrients contained in Moringa Oleifera it has all these nutrients in this 1 plant.

STROKE: A person that is experiencing a STROKE is deficient in such nutrients as: **Iron, Vitamin B12, Fiber, Vitamin D, Vitamin C, Folate and Antioxidants,** just to name a few. . But if you will notice from the list of nutrients contained in

Moringa Oleifera it has all these nutrients in this 1 plant.

ANEMIA: A person that is experiencing anemia is deficient in such nutrients as: **Iron, Vitamin B12, Folate, and Vitamin C,** just to name a few. . But if you will notice from the list of nutrients contained in Moringa Oleifera it has all these nutrients in this 1 plant.

So in reference to sickness and diseases in many cases **"It's A Deficiency In Vitamins and Minerals."** However, keep in mind as we close this chapter that not just any vitamin and mineral will do. The kinds that you find at the health food stores are mostly synthetic chemical based vitamins and minerals. These things are manufactured in a lab not grown by the Creator. Don't settle for second best when you can just as easily get it in its natural state from the hand of the Creator Himself. Moringa Oleifera is God's Superfood and triumphs all other herbs, vitamins and all other Superfoods.

6

Moringa Is A Food

"You know how your mother would tell you to eat your greens; she knew what was best for you and what your body needed."

Moringa Oleifera is an amazing plant that grows mainly in tropical and subtropical areas. This plant has been a staple of India for thousands of years and has been treated as both a food and a medicine in that region. Unlike many other superfoods it is a food plant with many medicinal uses and has the highest containment of nutritional value of any plant known. Singularly, Moringa Oleifera is a miracle plant that has so many benefits that it's almost unbelievable that one plant can do so much. I like to explain Moringa to individuals by saying, ***"when God made this tree he put in it exactly what our body needed in abundance."***

Also, the amazing thing about Moringa is that all parts of the tree can be used in various ways. Some of the many uses of this amazing tree are:

1. **A Natural Medicine**
2. **Water Purification**
3. **Food for Humans**
4. **Natural Pesticide**
5. **Food for Animals**
6. **Fertilizer**
7. **Etc....**

The various parts of the Moringa tree that is used in a variety of ways are:

1. **Fruit**
2. **Leaves**
3. **Seed**
4. **Flower**
5. **Branch**
6. **Root (be especially careful with the root, it's much stronger)**
7. **Bark**
8. **Oil**
9. **Drumstick or Seed Pods**
10. **Stems**
11. **Stalks**

12. Bark's Gum
13. Etc....

What an awesome plant created by an awesome Creator for the aid, help and assistance of mankind. However, in this book we have been and will focus on the food and medicinal aspect of Moringa Oleifera. Yes Moringa is actually a food, just like kale, spinach, collard greens, green beans, etc.... and in many places like Africa and India it has been used to fight malnutrition because of its abundant vitamin and mineral content.

Since Moringa is a food it can be treated just like any other food, it can be:

1. **Fried or steamed in any meal using the leaves.**
2. **Added in shakes.**
3. **Baked in goods.**
4. **The leaves can be eaten in a salad.**
5. **Used as a tea.**
6. **Added to beverages.**
7. **Used as a seasoning.**

8. The seeds can be eaten in small quantities just like sunflower seeds.
9. You can use the oil to cook with.
10. Put in coffee.
11. The powder can be sprinkled over salads, in oatmeal, smoothies, etc....
12. And hundreds of other ways...

Even though Moringa is a food just like spinach, kale, etc.... it's one of the only foods that you can eat and get a full day supply of nutrients. To streamline it even further Moringa also falls in the vegetable category and a food that's excellent for a vegetarian diet because it supplies for the vegan or vegetarian what they're missing in their daily nutrients.

So when you're thinking about a nutrient rich food to add to your next meal don't forget to include Moringa Oleifera in one of its many forms. Your body will think you in the way of prevention or restoration of health.

7

A New You Today, The Moringa Way

"Moringa Oleifera is God's Superfood, it's more than just a vitamin or mineral supplement, it's a way of life."

As we come to the conclusion of this book but we have not concluded all there is to know about Moringa Oleifera. This is a plant that God has created that is inexhaustible because of the continual unfolding revelation that is been revealed about what it can do for the human body.

When God created mankind from *"the dust of the ground"* Genesis 2:7 his body was whole and complete with nothing lacking and nothing missing. For the scripture says, *"And God saw everything that he had made, and, behold, it was very good."* Genesis 1:31a

But after the fall of man his body begins to deteriorate because man had disobeyed God in eating of the forbidden tree. God commanded him saying, *"Of every tree of the garden thou mayest freely eat: But of the tree of the knowledge of good and evil, thou shalt not eat of it: for in the day that thou eatest thereof thou shalt surely die."* Now we know that man did eat of the tree and physically he did not die immediately. However, he did die spiritually immediately for his spirit inwardly became dead towards God and his physical body followed suit many years later.

When God created man he was full of the life of God, he did not have eternal life but he had the breath of God in his being and he was really alive. It took Adam over 900 years to die physically because his physical body was permeating with the life of God and it had to learn how to die through deterioration. *"And all the days that Adam lived were nine hundred and thirty years and he died."* *Genesis 5:5* The body of Adam begin the process of becoming progressively worse. His health begin to decline, fail, collapse, drop and go on a downward slump until it had no more life in it. His once vibrant body began to descend from a higher level pulsating with life to a lower level of feebleness and eventually death.

Mankind has gone physically from been able to live to a ripe old age of 969 years old (Methuselah) to an age of merely 70 years if he's fortunate enough to live this long. His body has unfortunately deteriorated to the point that at times he/she only lives a few years in the case of children dying with diseases ravaging their bodies.

Mankind in this life will never see the days of 900 years ever again on this side of life, only during the 1000 year reign of Christ and when the new heaven and new earth is established. Nevertheless, we still need to take care of our temple which is our body to the best of our abilities. We need to take better care in the form of dietary, exercise and supplying our body with what it's deficient in on a daily basis.

Daily, you have all kinds of diseases and sicknesses that's pulling on your body and trying to invade your cells and enter your bloodstream to make you sick. Many times your body will fight off these things because God has created it to resist many foreign enemies that shouldn't enter it. However, when your body is deficient in the essential vitamins and minerals that's there to assist you these enemies will have a loophole and enter through an opening that's unprotected and lack resistance.

Many essential vitamins and minerals are there to aid, help and assist our bodies in the fight to protect us but when they're lacking the door is opened. Let's look at some essential vitamins and minerals that help protect and sustain our health and can keep us in tip top shape when they're operating in our body in abundance. Here are the essential vitamins:

1. *Vitamin A*

2. *Vitamin K*

3. *Vitamin D*

4. *Vitamin C*

5. *Vitamin E*

6. *Folate*

7. *Vitamin B6*

8. *Niacin*

9. *Riboflavin*

10. *Pantothenic Acid*

11. *Thiamin*

12. *Vitamin B12*

13. *Vitamin B Complex*

14. *Beta-Carotene*

15. Biotin

Here are the essential minerals:

1. Calcium
2. Potassium
3. Sodium
4. Magnesium
5. Phosphorus
6. Chloride
7. Trace Minerals
8. Boron
9. Chromium
10. Fluorine
11. Iodine
12. Iron
13. Manganese
14. Molybdenum

15. *Nickel*

16. *Selenium*

17. *Sulfur*

18. *Cobalt*

19. *Copper*

20. *Vanadium*

21. *Zinc*

All vitamins and minerals are necessary for the body to function at optimum but the ones listed above are especially necessary. The beauty of Moringa Oleifera is that all the essential vitamins and minerals are contained within this amazing plant. Since this superfood has come on the scene the day is now over that you will have to go to the store or order online various supplements to make sure that you have your adequate daily supply of vitamins and minerals. No longer will you have to spend hundreds of dollars for various supplements because Moringa has all the nutrients that your body requires in this 1 plant. It's time for a *"New You Today, The Moringa Way."* The product that we have labeled *"God's Superfood"* is ready to enhance your life and take your physical health to a new level of health and wellness.

It's your right as a human being to live your best life and how beneficial is life if you don't have the best of health? It's time to take responsibility for your own health, you only get one body therefore you must do all you can to preserve and sustain it in the best shape possible. It has been wisely stated that *"Your Health is Your Wealth"* for what good is wealth if you don't have the health to enjoy it?

Moringa Oleifera is truly an amazing and remarkable plant that God has created to assist you in your pursuit of good health for good health is God's highest wish for mankind. The word of God states, *"Beloved, I wish above all things that thou mayest prosper and be in health, even as thy soul prospereth."* 3 John 2 Right here the word of God shows you that God is interested in the whole man, spirit, soul and body. Not only is he interested but he has given us the remedy to help us fulfill the will of God for our lives in providing Moringa for our physical needs.

Are you ready for a ***"New You Today, The Moringa Way?"*** Then you need to become a partaker and not just a bystander of this amazing product and begin to reap the benefits of a Moringa induced life. The benefits you will derive physically are next to amazing as every organ of your body comes alive as you begin to take life into your body through Moringa Oleifera.

We have seen some truly amazing changes in the lives of individuals that have come into health and wellness through a daily consumption of this remarkable product. Many testimonies of changed lives, sustained lives and lives turned around. You do not have to remain in the state you're in; you can change your life if you're willing to shift from synthetic vitamins to the plant based and whole food supplements of Moringa Oleifera. From taking several different supplements a day to simply taking 1 supplement a day, Moringa Oleifera.

In this book we're handing you the physical blueprint to a changed life, this is a book that has the answers you're seeking for physical change. *Are you willing to try? Are you ready to try? Are you ready for a "New You Today, The Moringa Way"?*

The Greatest Plant on the Planet

Eden Wellness Moringa

123 N. Center Street

Goldsboro, NC 27530

www.edenwellnessmoringa.com

edenwellness@yahoo.com

These statements have not been evaluated by the Food & Drug Administration. This product information is not intended to diagnose, treat, cure or prevent any diseases.

The Greatest Plant on the Planet

The Greatest Plant on the Planet

The Greatest Plant on the Planet

The Greatest Plant on the Planet

The Greatest Plant on the Planet

www.ingramcontent.com/pod-product-compliance
Lightning Source LLC
Chambersburg PA
CBHW070030260726
48658CB00002B/567